Introduction

Dear Reader,

This book is for you. It's for every single mother navigating the often tumultuous waters of raising children alone. It's for those moments when you feel overwhelmed, exhausted, and uncertain of what the future holds. In these pages, you will find stories of perseverance, faith, and the unbreakable bond between a mother, her children, and the divine guidance that surrounds us all.

We are never truly alone. The love and help of God, coupled with the wisdom of our ancestors, especially those strong, loving grandmothers, are with us every step of the way. May these stories uplift your spirit and remind you that you are supported by a legacy of strength and love.

With love and light,

Jasmine

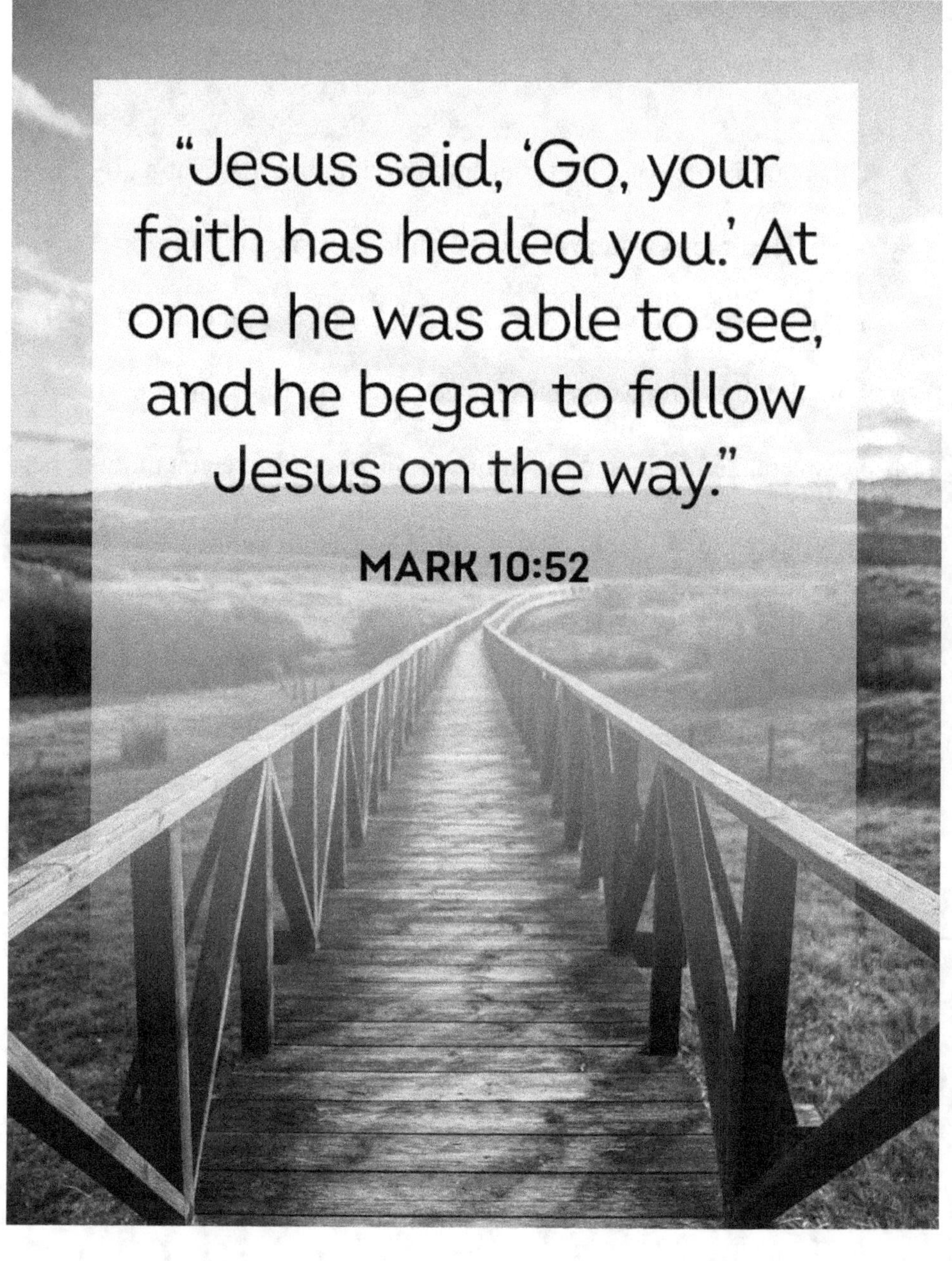
"Jesus said, 'Go, your faith has healed you.' At once he was able to see, and he began to follow Jesus on the way."

MARK 10:52

Chapter 1: The Weight of the World

Jessica sat in her small living room, the weight of the world on her shoulders. As a single mother of three young children, each day presented new challenges, and tonight was no different. Bills piled high on the kitchen counter, and the refrigerator was nearly empty. Yet, as the night settled in, Jessica found solace in a ritual that had become her lifeline: her evening prayers.

"Dear God," she whispered, tears streaming down her face, "I need your help. Guide me, show me the way. I can't do this alone."

A Legacy of Faith

Jessica's faith was not something new. It had been passed down through generations, rooted deeply in the wisdom and strength of her grandmother, Helen. Grandma Helen was a beacon of light, a woman of unwavering faith who believed in the power of prayer and the guidance of God. Even after her passing, Jessica felt her grandmother's presence, especially during her darkest moments.

Growing up, Jessica had spent countless hours in her grandmother's kitchen, listening to stories of resilience and miracles. Grandma

Helen would often say, "Child, there's nothing you can't overcome with faith and a little bit of grit. Remember, God and our ancestors are always with you."

The Struggle

After her divorce, Jessica found herself struggling to make ends meet. Her job as a part-time cashier barely covered the essentials, and the prospect of finding better employment seemed daunting with three children to care for. Each day felt like an uphill battle, but giving up was not an option. Her children depended on her, and she was determined to provide them with a stable and loving home.

Despite her efforts, the financial strain grew heavier. Jessica knew she needed more than just a miracle; she needed a plan. She remembered her grandmother's words, "God helps those who help themselves. Keep your faith strong and your mind sharp."

A Turning Point

One evening, as Jessica was tucking her children into bed, her oldest daughter, Mia, handed her a small, worn-out Bible that had belonged to Grandma Helen. "Mommy," Mia said, "Grandma always said to read this when you need help."

Jessica took the Bible, feeling a wave of comfort wash over her. She opened it to a random page and began to read. Her eyes fell upon a passage from Matthew 7:7-8: "Ask, and it will be given to you; seek, and you will find; knock, and the door will be opened to you."

Inspired, Jessica decided to take action. She spent the next few weeks updating her resume, applying for jobs, and seeking assistance from local community resources. She also joined a support group for single mothers at her church, where she found camaraderie and practical advice.

The Miracle

One morning, as Jessica was dropping Mia off at school, she received a phone call that changed everything. A local nonprofit organization was looking for a program coordinator, and her resume had stood out. The job offered a substantial salary increase and benefits that included childcare assistance.

Jessica couldn't believe it. She remembered her prayers and her grandmother's words. With tears of joy, she accepted the position, feeling a renewed sense of hope and purpose.

A New Beginning

The new job not only improved Jessica's financial situation but also allowed her to help other struggling families. She used her own experiences to inspire and uplift others, becoming a beacon of hope within her community.

Jessica's journey was far from over, but she knew she was not alone. She carried with her the love and guidance of God and her grandmother, whose spirit remained a constant source of strength. Each night, she continued her prayers, thanking God for His blessings and asking for continued guidance.

Jessica's story is a testament to the power of faith, resilience, and the enduring love of our ancestors. It reminds us that no matter how difficult our circumstances, we can find strength in the legacy of those who came before us and in the unwavering belief that we are never truly alone.

As you embark on your journey as a single mother, remember Jessica's story. Embrace your faith, seek out community, and never underestimate the power of prayer and determination. Your challenges may seem insurmountable at times, but with God's love and the strength of your ancestors, you can overcome them. You are part of a legacy of resilience and love, and your story, too, will inspire future generations.

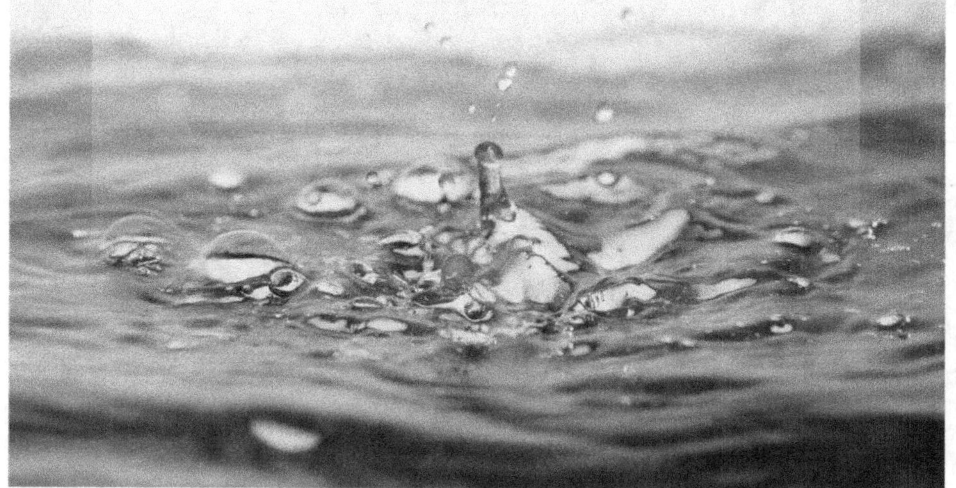

"Trust in the Lord with all your heart; don't rely on your own intelligence. Know him in all your paths, and he will keep your ways straight."

PROVERBS 3:5-6

Chapter 2: The Power of Faith

Tiana stood in the kitchen, staring at the pile of dirty dishes in the sink. The sound of her twin boys, Jackson and Jordan, playing in the living room brought a small smile to her face, but the exhaustion in her bones was undeniable. As a single mother working two jobs, Tiana knew the meaning of hard work and sacrifice. Her journey was one of relentless perseverance, but also one of deep faith and spiritual guidance.

A Mother's Sacrifice

Tiana's life took a dramatic turn when her husband left, leaving her to care for their two boys alone. The shock and betrayal were overwhelming, but she had no choice but to keep moving forward. With her family's support and the wisdom of her mother, Lorraine, Tiana began to piece her life back together.

Growing up, Tiana often heard her mother say, "Tiana, life isn't always fair, but God never gives us more than we can handle. You come from a long line of strong women, and we don't break—we bend." These words echoed in her mind as she navigated the challenges of single motherhood.

The Struggle

Balancing two jobs as a waitress and a part-time office assistant left Tiana with little time for anything else. She missed the days when she could sit and read bedtime stories to her boys, help them with their homework, or simply enjoy their laughter without the looming stress of bills and deadlines. The financial strain was a constant burden, but Tiana was determined to provide for her children and give them the life they deserved.

Despite her efforts, the reality of their situation weighed heavily on Tiana. There were days when she questioned if she was doing enough, if she was strong enough. Yet, every night, as she put her boys to bed, she whispered a prayer, asking for strength, guidance, and the courage to keep going.

A Moment of Desperation

One particularly difficult evening, after a long day at work and with the boys finally asleep, Tiana collapsed on the couch, tears streaming down her face. The weight of her responsibilities felt unbearable, and she cried out in desperation, "God, I don't know if I can do this anymore. I need your help."

In that moment of vulnerability, Tiana felt a presence, a warmth that enveloped her. She remembered the stories her mother told her about their ancestors, women who had faced incredible hardships and yet had found the strength to persevere. Lorraine often spoke of her own grandmother, Evelyn, who raised seven children on her own during the Great Depression. "Grandma Evelyn always said, 'When you feel like you can't go on, remember that you carry the strength of those who came before you. You're never alone.'"

A Turning Point

The next day, with a renewed sense of purpose, Tiana decided to make a change. She began looking for better job opportunities, determined to find something that would allow her to spend more time with her children while providing for their needs. She reached out to community organizations for support and took advantage of resources she had previously overlooked.

One afternoon, while attending a local job fair, Tiana met a woman named Angela, who worked for a nonprofit organization that helped single mothers find employment and provided access to affordable childcare. Angela was moved by Tiana's story and offered to help her update her resume and connect her with potential employers.

The Miracle

A few weeks later, Tiana received a call from a local community center looking for a program coordinator for their after-school activities. The position offered a decent salary, benefits, and most importantly, a schedule that would allow her to spend evenings with her boys. Overwhelmed with gratitude, Tiana accepted the job.

The new role not only improved their financial situation but also allowed Tiana to be more present in her children's lives. She found joy in her work, helping other families and creating a supportive community. Her boys thrived, knowing their mother was always there for them.

A New Beginning

Tiana's journey was far from over, but she faced each day with a newfound strength and faith. She knew that she was not alone, that the love and guidance of her ancestors and the presence of God were with her every step of the way. Each night, as she tucked Jackson and Jordan into bed, she whispered a prayer of gratitude and asked for continued strength and guidance.

Tiana's story is a powerful reminder of the resilience and strength that lies within us all. It is a testament to the enduring love of our ancestors and the unshakeable faith that can carry us through even the darkest of times.

As you read Tiana's story, may you find inspiration and hope. Remember that you are never alone in your struggles. You carry within you the legacy of those who came before, and with faith and determination, you can overcome any obstacle. Let Tiana's journey be a beacon of light, guiding you through your own challenges and reminding you of the strength and love that surrounds you.

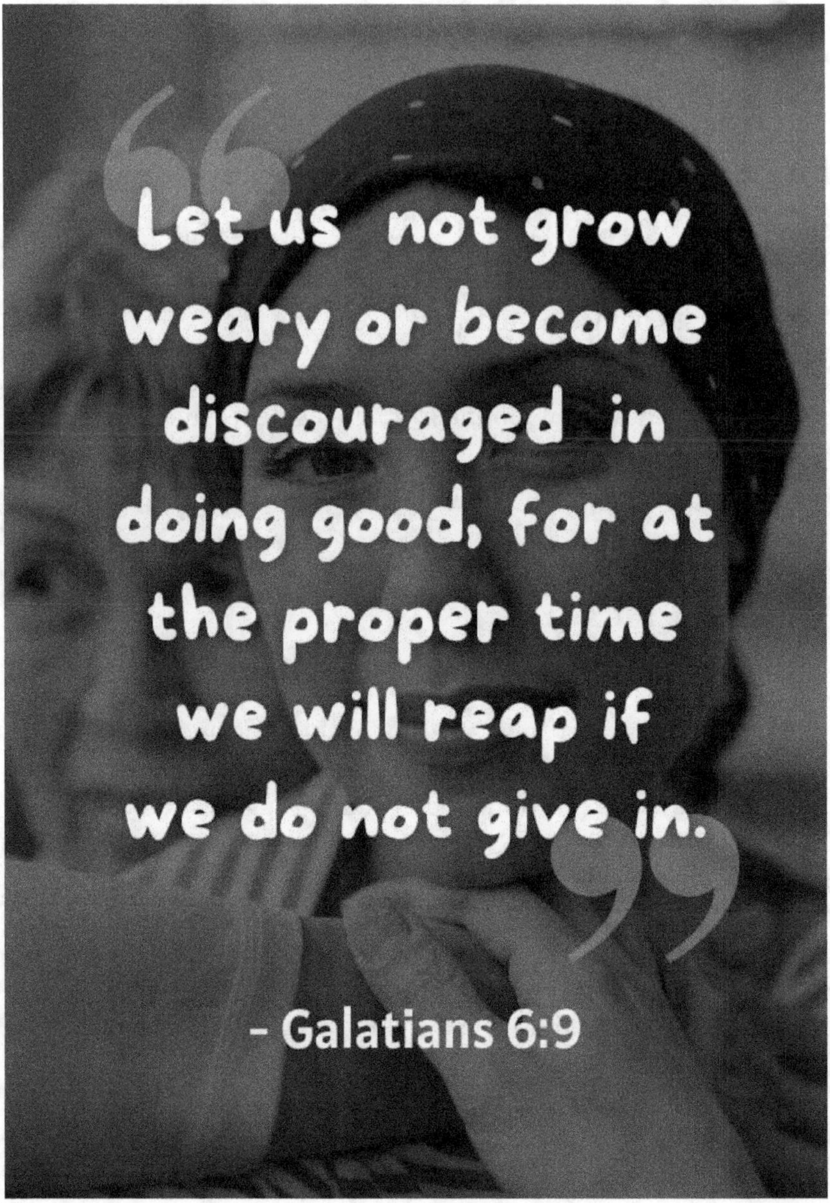

Let us not grow
weary or become
discouraged in
doing good, for at
the proper time
we will reap if
we do not give in.

- Galatians 6:9

Chapter 3: The Strength Within

Tanya's life had been a whirlwind of challenges, but nothing compared to the decision to leave an abusive relationship. It was a leap into the unknown, driven by a fierce determination to protect her daughter, Lily. The road ahead was uncertain, but Tanya was resolute in her quest for a better life.

The Decision to Leave

Leaving was the hardest part. Tanya had endured years of emotional and physical abuse, feeling trapped and isolated. But the turning point came one night when Lily, barely four years old, witnessed an altercation. Seeing the fear in her daughter's eyes gave Tanya the strength she needed. She packed a small bag with essentials, took Lily by the hand, and left the only home she had known for years.

A New Beginning

With no job and limited resources, Tanya found herself in a city that felt both promising and daunting. The first few nights were spent in a cheap motel, the money she had saved quickly dwindling. Tanya's mind raced with fears and doubts, but she clung to the memories of her grandmother, whose resilience had always been a source of inspiration.

The Dream

One particularly restless night, Tanya dreamt of her grandmother. In the dream, her grandmother's hands—weathered yet gentle—held hers firmly. She whispered words of encouragement, telling Tanya that strength and courage were already within her. She woke up with a renewed sense of purpose and a feeling of comfort, as if her grandmother was watching over her.

Reaching Out

The next morning, Tanya took a courageous step. She reached out to a women's shelter. The shelter provided immediate refuge and connected her with resources to help her get back on her feet. The staff at the shelter were compassionate and understanding, offering Tanya and Lily a safe place to stay and the emotional support they desperately needed.

Finding Stability

Tanya's journey was far from easy, but she faced each day with determination. She found a job at a local grocery store, working long hours to save money. Despite the exhaustion, Tanya enrolled in night classes, determined to build a future for herself and Lily. Her grandmother's stories of resilience played in her mind, reminding her that she was capable of overcoming any obstacle.

Building a Home

Slowly but surely, Tanya began to create a stable, loving home for Lily. She found a small apartment and filled it with second-hand furniture and decorations. The most important addition was the warmth and love she infused into their new home. Every night, she read to Lily, telling her stories of strong women, including her great-grandmother.

Discovering Inner Strength

Tanya realized that her grandmother's strength had always been within her. The courage to leave, the determination to provide for her daughter, and the resilience to face each challenge were all part of her legacy. Tanya's journey was a testament to the power of inner strength and the support of those who believe in us.

Tanya's story is a powerful reminder that we all possess the strength within to overcome life's toughest challenges. Her journey from an abusive relationship to creating a loving home for Lily illustrates the transformative power of courage and resilience. As Tanya built a new life, she discovered that the strength she needed had always been inside her, guided by the love and wisdom of her grandmother.

May Tanya's story inspire you to find your own inner strength and remind you that, no matter the obstacles, you have the power to create a better future for yourself and your loved ones. Trust in your journey and the support of those who care for you, and know that you are never truly alone.

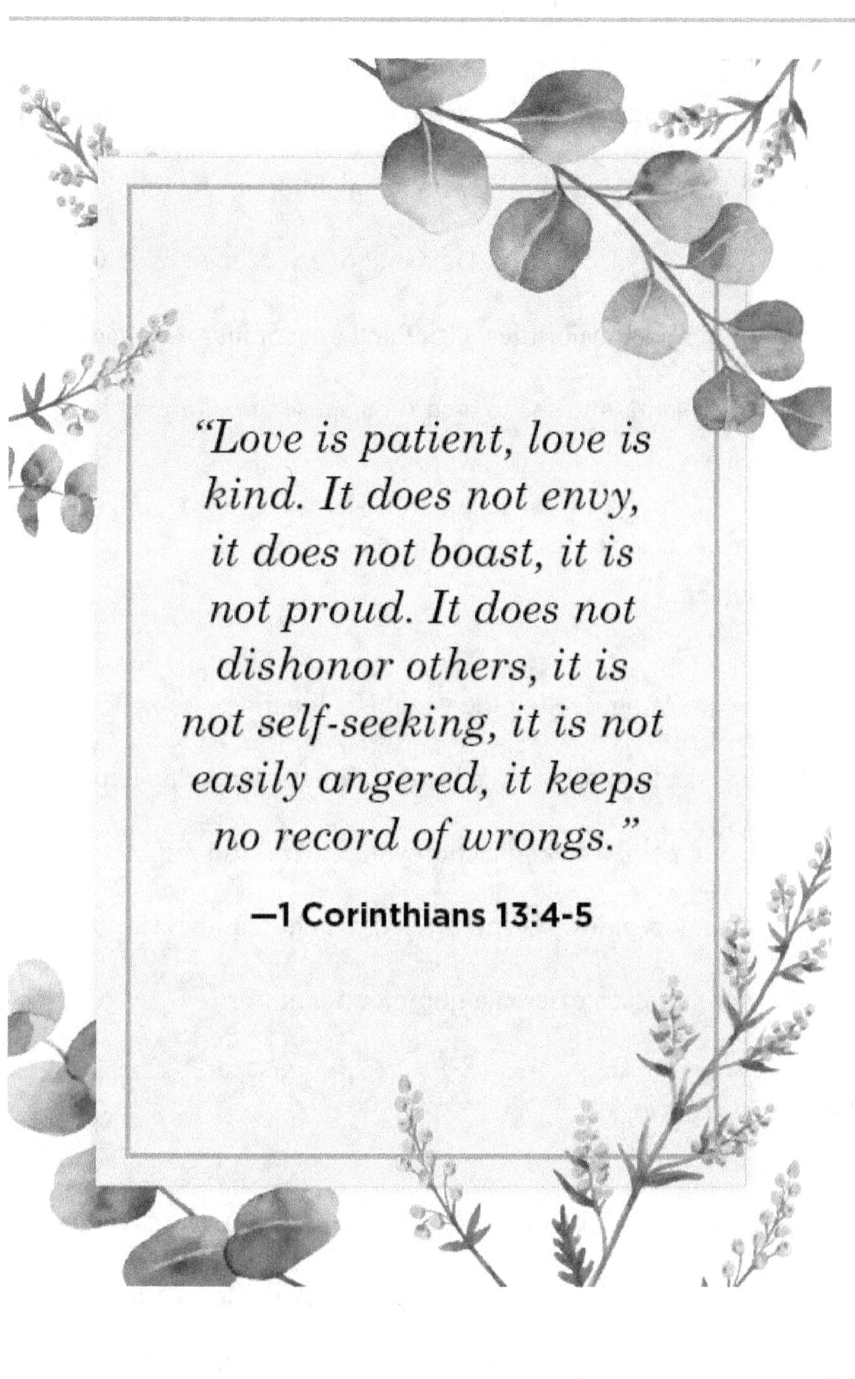

"Love is patient, love is kind. It does not envy, it does not boast, it is not proud. It does not dishonor others, it is not self-seeking, it is not easily angered, it keeps no record of wrongs."

—1 Corinthians 13:4-5

Chapter 4: A Community of Love

Simone's life was turned upside down after the sudden passing of her husband. As a single mother of two young children, she found herself in a new city, feeling isolated and overwhelmed by the enormity of her responsibilities. Grief and uncertainty weighed heavily on her heart, and she longed for a sense of belonging and support.

Seeking Solace

One Sunday morning, feeling the weight of loneliness more than ever, Simone decided to attend a local church service. She hoped to find solace and perhaps a connection with others who might understand her struggles. As she entered the church, the warmth and tranquility of the place offered a glimmer of comfort.

Meeting Margaret

After the service, Simone lingered in the church courtyard, watching families and friends chat and laugh together. An older woman approached her with a gentle smile. "Hello, dear," she said, introducing herself as Margaret. There was something about Margaret that reminded Simone of her grandmother—the same kindness in her eyes and the same comforting presence.

A New Friendship

Margaret struck up a conversation with Simone, asking about her children and how she was settling into the new city. Simone found herself opening up about her recent loss and the challenges she faced as a single mother. Margaret listened with empathy and shared her own experiences of overcoming hardships.

Margaret invited Simone to join her for coffee after the next service. Simone accepted, and over the next few weeks, their friendship blossomed. Margaret's wisdom, support, and unwavering kindness provided Simone with the strength she desperately needed.

Introducing the Network

Margaret introduced Simone to a network of single mothers within the church. These women, like Simone, had faced various challenges and were raising their children on their own. They met regularly for support, sharing their experiences, advice, and encouragement.

At the first meeting, Simone was struck by the openness and camaraderie among the women. They discussed everything from parenting tips to job opportunities, offering practical help and emotional support. Simone realized she was not alone in her struggles, and this community of strong, resilient women quickly became her lifeline.

Finding Strength in Community

Through her involvement with this network, Simone began to regain her confidence and sense of purpose. The other mothers shared their own stories of triumph over adversity, inspiring Simone to keep moving forward. She saw firsthand how God works through people, placing angels in our lives when we need them the most.

Margaret, in particular, became a guiding light for Simone. She was always there with a listening ear, a word of advice, or a shoulder to cry on. Margaret's own story of loss and recovery served as a powerful reminder that it was possible to rebuild a life filled with love and joy.

Creating an Extended Family

Simone's children also benefited from this newfound community. They made friends with other children who understood what it was like to grow up in a single-parent household. Church gatherings, picnics, and playdates became regular events, providing a sense of stability and happiness for her children.

Margaret and the other mothers became Simone's extended family. They celebrated birthdays, supported each other through difficult times, and created a network of love and support that was invaluable. Simone found herself thriving in ways she had never imagined possible when she first moved to the city.

Simone's journey from isolation and grief to finding a supportive community highlights the importance of reaching out and allowing others into our lives. Her story illustrates that love and support can come from unexpected places and that God often works through the people around us.

The community of single mothers, led by the compassionate and wise Margaret, became Simone's sanctuary. Through their collective strength, shared experiences, and unwavering support, Simone discovered a renewed sense of hope and belonging. She learned that while the journey may be challenging, the love and guidance of others can light the way forward.

May Simone's story inspire you to seek out and embrace the support of those around you, and to recognize the angels that God places in your life. No matter the difficulties you face, remember that a community of love and support is never far away.

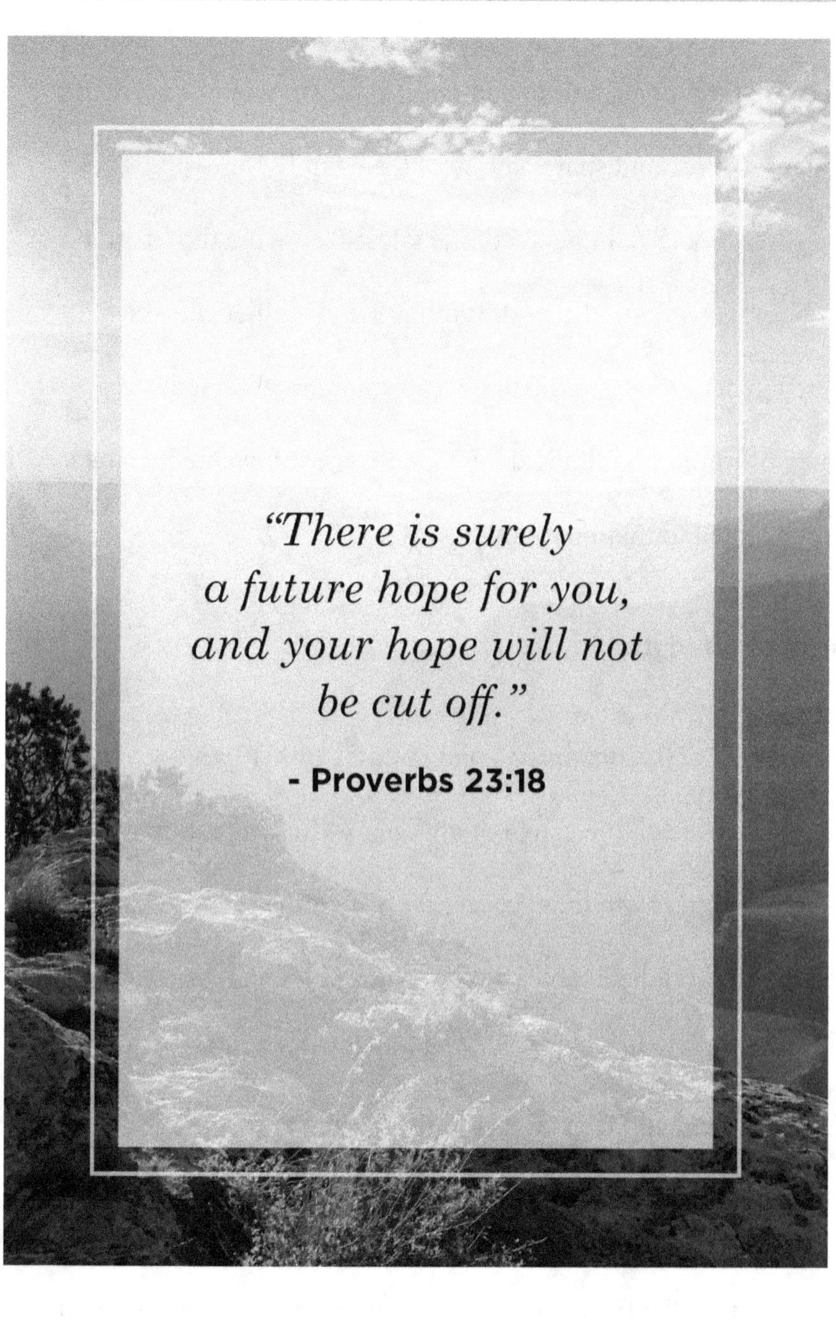

"There is surely
a future hope for you,
and your hope will not
be cut off."

- Proverbs 23:18

Chapter 5: The Legacy of Love

In the quiet moments before bedtime, Aahliyah would sit with her daughter, Chloe, and share stories of their family's history. These stories were more than just bedtime tales; they were the lifeblood of their heritage, a reminder of the strength and resilience passed down through generations. Aahliyah's great-grandmother had been a woman of immense faith and love, and Aahliyah wanted Chloe to feel connected to that powerful legacy.

Stories of Strength

Each night, Aahliyah painted vivid pictures of her great-grandmother's life. She spoke of a woman who had endured the harshest of times with unwavering faith, a woman whose hands had tilled the soil, cradled babies, and wiped away countless tears. Aahliyah's stories were filled with the trials and triumphs of a matriarch who had faced adversity with grace and courage.

One story that Chloe loved was about her great-grandmother's journey during the Great Migration, moving from the rural South to the bustling North in search of better opportunities. Despite the challenges of starting over in a new place, she remained steadfast in her faith and determination, carving out a new life for her family.

Chloe's Question

One evening, as they were wrapping up another story, Chloe looked up at her mother with wide, curious eyes. "Mommy, how do you stay so strong?" she asked, her voice filled with wonder.

Aahliyah smiled warmly, her heart swelling with love for her inquisitive daughter. She took Chloe's small hands in her own and said, "I have the love of God, and the hands of our ancestors guiding me." She explained that their family had always relied on faith and the wisdom of those who came before them.

The Power of Ancestral Guidance

Aahliyah told Chloe that they were never truly alone. Even in the darkest moments, the strength of their grandmothers lived on within them. This spiritual connection was a source of immense comfort and power, reminding them that they were part of something much larger than themselves.

She shared how, during her own difficult times, she would close her eyes and imagine her great-grandmother standing beside her, offering silent support. This visualization helped Aahliyah feel grounded and resilient, knowing that the love and guidance of her ancestors were always present.

Building a Foundation of Faith

Aahliyah's words resonated deeply with Chloe. From that night forward, Chloe carried the stories and lessons of her ancestors in her heart. She understood that she, too, had the power and support of a legacy filled with strong, loving women.

This legacy of love and faith became the foundation of their family. It was a wellspring of hope and courage that they could draw from whenever life presented its inevitable challenges. Aahliyah continued to nurture this connection through their nightly stories, ensuring that Chloe would always feel the presence and strength of their ancestors.

A Living Legacy

As Chloe grew older, she began to share the stories with others, keeping the legacy alive. She spoke of her great-grandmother's resilience, her mother's unwavering faith, and the enduring love that connected them all. These stories inspired her friends and peers, spreading the message of hope and strength even further.

Chloe realized that her family's legacy was not just about the past but also about the future. It was about living in a way that honored the strength and love of those who came before them, and about passing on that wisdom to the next generation.

The legacy of love and faith handed down through Aahliyah's family became a guiding light for both her and Chloe. It was a reminder that no matter what challenges they faced, they were never alone. They had the love of God and the strength of their ancestors to carry them through.

May Aahliyah and Chloe's story inspire you to embrace your own heritage and find strength in the love and wisdom of those who came before you. Remember that you are part of a legacy that can

empower you to face life's challenges with grace and courage.

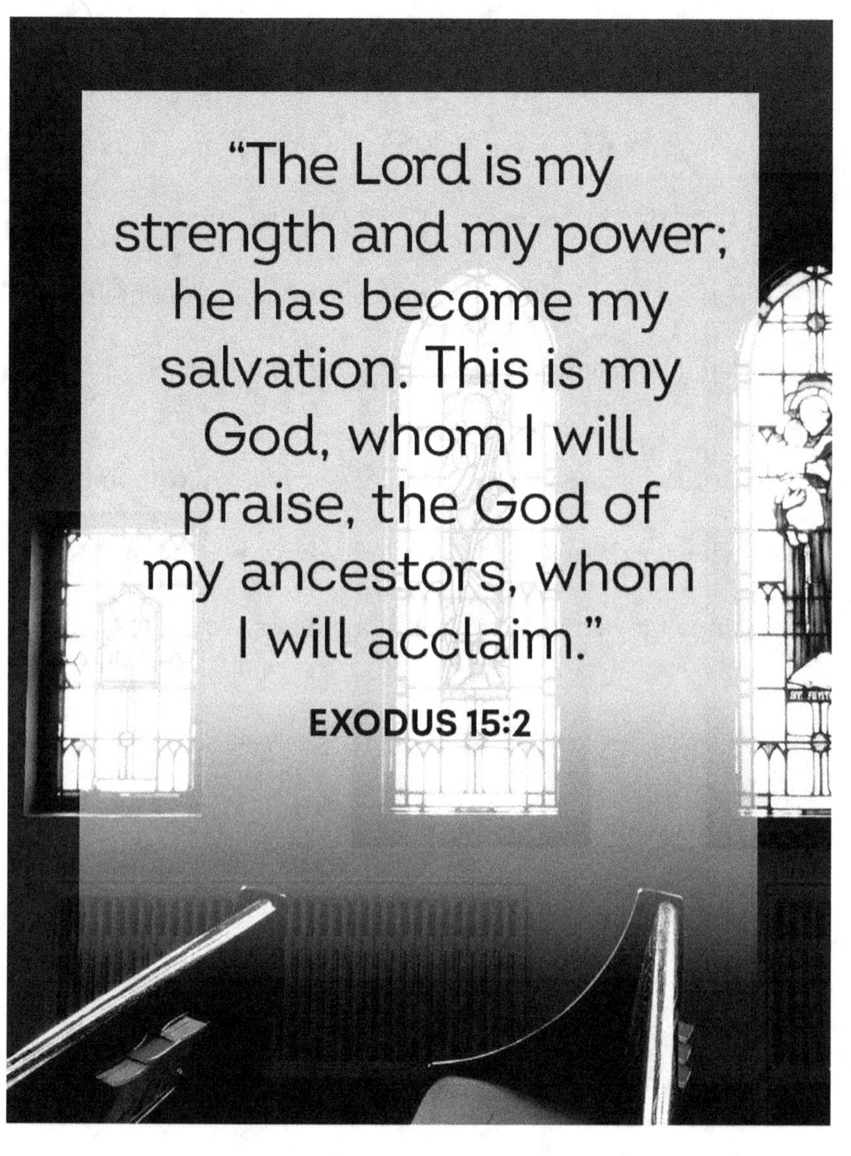
"The Lord is my strength and my power; he has become my salvation. This is my God, whom I will praise, the God of my ancestors, whom I will acclaim."

EXODUS 15:2

Conclusion

To all the single mothers reading this book, remember that you are not alone. You carry within you the strength of your ancestors and the love of God. In your moments of doubt and fear, reach out to this divine support system. Trust in the guidance of your grandmothers, and know that their hands are always there to lift you up.

May these stories inspire you to embrace your journey with faith, love, and resilience. You are stronger than you know, and your story is a testament to the incredible power of a mother's love.

With all my heart,

A single mother and her son,

Jasmine McKinney and Kurell David